Walking For Good Health

A Comprehensive Guide To Good Health Just By Walking!!!

By

Natalie Johnson

Table Of Contents

Introduction

I want to thank you and congratulate you for downloading the book, *Walking For Good Health: A Comprehensive Guide To Good Health Just By Walking!!!*

This book contains proven steps and strategies on how a simple thing such as walking could become one of your most powerful tools for good health.

When babies start making their precious first steps, virtually everyone becomes overjoyed. Mothers, fathers, grandparents, even friends and extended family members delight at the milestone their wonderful bundle of joy had just reached. Pictures are taken, videos are recorded, messages of triumph are sent—"My baby's walking!"

If walking is something that is incredibly important, you would not know of it from then on. While babies are praised and encouraged to walk, adults whine and sigh inwardly at the prospect of walking a few blocks to go to school, to work, or to pick up their laundry at the local cleaners. People invented round feet to do the walking for them—wheels on bicycles, motorbikes, cars, and all sorts of automobiles used in public transport. It seems that everybody has forgotten the joys they had when they first walked, and now even more so! People have thus invented door-to-door deliveries, so that you would not even have to get on your bike, car, or the bus. People have come to the point when even the thought of standing up from the couch or the computer makes them whine and sigh.

This book will bring back all the glory that comes with walking that has been lost through the ages. In a world with so many complex diseases and conditions now plague mankind, requiring so many complicated modes of treatment, it seems oddly humbling to know that something as simple as putting one foot forward after another is the answer to good health. May this book enlighten you in ways that most of society seems to have forgotten!

Thanks again for downloading this book, I hope you enjoy it!

Chapter 1

The Dangers of Being Sedentary

You might have heard the word before, once, twice, or many times over. *Sedentary*. It is a popular word most often followed by the word *lifestyle*, and most usually used to shortly explain a whole host of complications and diseases that burden man. Diabetes. Obesity. Cardiovascular disease. And yes, even cancer.

Sedentary means *to stay in one place*. This would mean that a sedentary lifestyle would mean living in one place for a lengthy period, probably a lifetime. But then again, how could living in one place be a cause of so many diseases? That cannot be right – we are no longer living in the Stone Age when men had to roam the wilds and shake the soil from their bare feet in search of food and shelter. Food and shelter have become more sustainable these days.

But *sedentary lifestyle* is not as such. Speaking of soil being shaken from bare feet, *sedentary* is also used to describe *soil*, and *sedentary soil* refers to the deeper part of soil layers that more or less does not budge from its place.

This is the kind of lifestyle that invites diabetes, obesity, and all the other big words mentioned above – a lifestyle where one hardly budges from sitting or lying down.

It does not matter if you stay in one place for your whole life—as long as you do not live and die sitting on a chair. A sedentary lifestyle is one that involves little to no physical activity, or that the only physical activities involved are those when you stretch out your hand to reach the remote and jab your finger onto the buttons. It is a lifestyle where you get up from bed to sit for an hour at the breakfast table, sit for a quarter of an hour in your car, sit in your office for a good 6-8 hours, then go home to sit for a few more hours at the dinner table then in front of the TV. It is a lifestyle that cycles around little variations of that, day in and day out.

Why it has to Stop
Sitting is the new smoking, says scientists and medical professionals everywhere. It might not seem much, until you remember that *smoking kills*. In fact, smoking is the kind of killer that tends to kill you slowly, feeding you an addictive feeling of false comfort until it strikes at your throat (or more to the point, your lungs) at the end. By that time, most of the battle has already been lost, wasted away on years

2

when you thought another stick of cigarette is just that – another stick of cigarette.

But how could another hour of sitting down be more than just another hour of sitting down? Sitting is comfortable, sitting relieves tension from the feet and legs, and, more importantly, sitting is when you can be your most productive as you type away at your keyboards or to scribble onto your notes. How could that be so bad?

Oh, let us count the ways.

In recent studies, prolonged sitting has been attributed to a huge factor in the development of cardiovascular diseases, obesity, and diabetes – all the big words mentioned earlier. This is because sitting down, especially sitting down for hours at a time, sends a signal to the brain that the body is not just resting, but is hibernating, just as in deep sleep. This in turn makes the brain fire signals for the body to decrease its metabolic functions, which would then trigger a chain reaction that includes an increase in the blood's cholesterol level, a decrease in the blood's HDL or "good" cholesterol level, and an increase to the body's insensitivity to insulin. Just as every puff of cigar smoke accumulates more tar and more nicotine in your system, every hour of sitting down adds fat, sugar, and sludge in your system until it kills you.

Make no mistake about it: prolonged sitting *can* kill you.

In a study conducted by Australia's Sax Institute[1] involving at least 200,000 people aged 45 and above and are of different physical states, genders, and statuses, it was shown that a person who sits at an average of 11 hours a day were likely to die within the next three years by up to 40%. This is regardless of physical states, meaning the study included smokers, diabetics, normal people, doctors, runners, athletes, single moms, ordinary office workers—everyone. It does not matter if you are physically fit or already on your deathbed. Sitting down for up to 11 hours a day or more will likely kill you within the next three years.

The results astounded the researchers, yet it also alarmed them, all the more so because all the other studies are correlating to the findings of the Sax Institute research. In a separate study conducted by *BMJ Open* in the US[2], for instance, it was stated that sitting for 3 hours every day takes two years off a person's lifespan. That is just in sitting *for three hours.* How much more if you sit for more than 3 hours a day? Think about how many hours you spend sitting down in school or at the office, and how many more when you watch the TV at home.

Truly, these statistics are a cause for concern. Ask any ordinary employee and you will know why—most of us spend all our days cooped up in an office, hunched over the keyboards, sitting inside a cramped cubicle space. The only walking these people ever do is to get water or coffee and to go to the bathroom. No wonder professionals were so alarmed.

But sometimes, the most alarming of problems only require the simplest of solutions. The only way to combat prolonged sitting is to keep moving – to keep walking.

Chapter 2:

Why Walk?

Why not? It might come off as a stupid answer to you, but set that aside for a moment and think deeply about the answer. Why not? The One who engineered the human body has seen fit to grace humans with two feet, sturdy legs, and powerful thighs, so why not use them? Why should you require beta blockers to heal your heart, statins to lower your cholesterol, metformin and insulin to manage your diabetes, when your legs and feet could do so for free? The answer will then seem a bit clearer, will it not? Why not, indeed?

Benefits of Walking

Do a quick Google search about the benefits of walking and you will not come out short. A slow stroll is therapeutic for the body and the mind, especially to older patients. A brisk morning walk is a good form of daily exercise to keep the heart and lungs in tip-top shape. Walking with therapeutic shoes or sandals—the ones with the rounded knobs you can find in most Asian stores—are known to alleviate symptoms or problems of internal organs. Walking with bare feet on grass, mud, dry earth, or on the wet sand submerged under seawater are all known to cause benefits to the body. Walking is beneficial to the body!

In as much as the same that sitting down sends signals to the body to slow down its metabolic function, walking sends signals to the body to speed up its metabolic function. This means the body will actively nourish muscles instead of shutting down everything as it does during hibernation. This means the body will break down fat to use as energy as opposed to store it for the long winter. All of these and more are caused by a simple movement of the legs.

In fact, a part of an occupational therapist's job is to make sure bedridden patients get their share of walking, or something similar to it. Even patients in a coma—people who are dead to the world, without power to move their limbs freely—have to be physically ambulated daily, so that their brains will know that their bodies are still active and will still need nourishment. What happens when a patient does not move from his or her position for a long time? A lot of ugly things, such as muscle wasting, muscle weakness, and bed sores.

This is because the legs act as pistons, helping the heart to pump up oxygen and nutrient-rich blood throughout the body, and also to return used blood back up to the lungs and heart. The heart is situated high up on a vertical person, and even as a strong knuckle-sized hardy muscle, the heart cannot pump itself to death so that the blood will reach the tips of your toes.

Ever wonder why some people have varicose veins? Varicose veins are long, spidery, bulging veins that adorn the backs of the knees, or even down on the legs and on the lower abdomen. These are because veins have no valves that will push blood back up to the heart, so people who stand up or sit down for prolonged periods will have blood pooling at their legs. This pressure causes the delicate veins to rupture, causing the spidery look so often abhorred by women who like to show off their long legs.

It does not happen just to the legs. Even if a person was lying down, the heart is not strong enough to pump blood for it to reach until the far ends of the appendages. All blood will pool along his or her back, causing pressure against the mattress, and later on, festering bed sores.

Aside from such, the calf and thigh muscles are broken down from misuse. Even asleep, the body's internal organs still work to a degree, and will require nourishment. Protein—muscle—is easier to break down than fat, and if the muscles of the leg are not in use...

Walking prevents all of these and more. With just the simple motion of moving your feet, blood that has pooled on the bottom is forcefully pushed back up into the upper veins, to where the heart could easily pump it back into flow. Walking will also engage the muscles along the calf, thigh, abdomen, and buttocks so no muscle wastage occurs. Also, as your body becomes aware that you are active, it will refrain from breaking down protein for energy, and will break down fat instead.

Pressure Points

In Eastern medicine, it has long been believed that the soles of the feet are connected to different organs or body parts, and that massaging these points by putting pressure on them will also heal the connecting body parts.

Reflexology is one such practice that believes in this ideology. They even have maps to show which organs or body parts certain points on the left and right soles are connected. Reflexologists use wooden sticks with blunted ends to put pressure onto these points during therapy.

Those who do not have the leisure to be seen by a reflexologist could still experience the treatment by getting one of the many variants of therapeutic sandals or shoes. These have knobby points made from wood or strong plastic along the sole, so walking in them will put pressure on the points with each step.

There are therapeutic spas that even use hot stones for therapy. They usually have cobbled paths or walkways of smooth stones that have been lit by warm sunlight, with customers walking barefoot along them. The hot stones provide heat and pressure to the soles of the feet and their pressure points.

Leeching of Toxins

Aside from exercise and therapeutic benefits, walking—especially walking barefoot in seawater—is also said to be incredibly powerful in leeching toxins from the body. Alternative medicine practitioners call this as *Thalassotherapy,* in which they believe that the ocean's salt and mineral-rich waters, along with its warm temperature and climate, are beneficial in expelling the body's toxins and free radicals.

The soles of the feet, aside from having pressure points, are also believed to be a door of sorts, in the same way as mouths, noses, ears, and eyes are. As they are situated at the bottommost part of the body, most of the toxins along with the blood pool on them. Advocates of thalassotherapy claim that walking along the sandy beach, or better if the feet were submerged under seawater, will not only condition the cardiovascular system, but will also help in releasing the toxins accumulated in the body.

Of Science and Skepticism
It is quite understandable if you should be a bit skeptic about pressure points and about leeching toxins. Most western doctors will wrinkle their noses at the idea, and with reason—that is not part of what they have learned in all of their years of study and practice. Alternative medicine practitioners will swear their efficacy; western medical professionals will not.

Much of these will seem too farfetched to skeptics, but even science agrees that walking is extremely beneficial to the body. Ask anyone, whether they are medical practitioners from the east or from the west, and they will all agree that walking is a wonderful activity that will do nothing but good. It is an activity so simple that two year-olds could even do... you would not want to be beaten by a two year-old, would you?

"Two year olds don't have 9-5 desk jobs," you might mutter sourly, but you do have a valid point. This same point was raised by many researchers, all of whom were alarmed at the detrimental effects of sitting still. But with so many jobs requiring workers to sit still throughout the day, what is there to do?

Science has the answer. Science and invention. Walking is such an invaluable exercise that people have invented—and have implemented—what is known as the treadmill desk, which is exactly what it sounds like – a treadmill attacked to a desk where you can do your work. Many offices across the US, UK, and Canada have tried getting one or two, for their employees who would like to try walking while working.

This is the reason why walking is preferred to running. Even at a very slow pace, walking burns calories, increases the metabolism, and works out the muscles. It might not burn as much calories as a 15-minute jog, but if you have the rest of the day to walk the miles while typing on your laptop or answering calls, you honestly will not notice the difference – but you will certainly notice the improvement in your health.

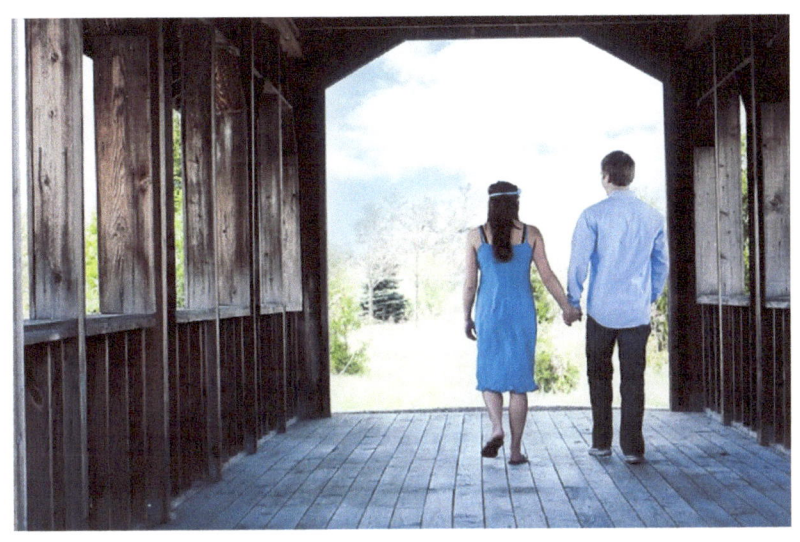

Chapter 3:
Early Morning Stroll

So you have learned why you should walk, now you might question *when* the best time it is to walk, especially if you plan on walking outside. An easy answer would be "anytime", and, really, exercise should not be put aside just because it is way past its best time, but there is a certain time when walking outdoors is more beneficial than during most, and that is early in the morning.

Depending on where you are, this is the time around 6-10 am, when the sun has risen but is not too hot as to cause sunburns. Some areas receive stronger sunlight than others, such as Florida and California and the tropics in Asia, while some can enjoy later hours under mild sunlight.

But why is sunlight so beneficial? In a recent study, it was found that the reason most people who work the night oil, the graveyard shifts, or plainly during the night are overweight or obese is because they lack exposure to sunlight. Sunlight is necessary for the body to synthesize vitamin D, which, as it turns out, regulates a person's hunger and satiety hormone, among other things.

Have you ever wondered why you always seem hungry when you always stay up late, or when you always work or study through the night? That is due to the lack of vitamin D in your system. Yes, we can get vitamin D from the foods that we eat or from supplements, but without the precursor found in sunlight, the body will not be able to synthesize it, meaning the body will not be able to use it. There is a reason why the media portray computer or video game geeks as obese, unkempt people who shut themselves in the dark in their parents' house's basement—people who lack exposure to sunlight have no control to their satiety levels, meaning once they go hungry, they will eat and eat, without feeling full. Once they *do* feel sated, they are well past they satiety levels, with all the calories they have been eating going to their thighs, buttocks, belly—everywhere. It would be wishful thinking to say that these people wolf down on plates of fresh greens or lightly steamed veggies, but we all know it is the bag of chips or the pint of ice cream that they reach for.

Walking is an exercise that aids in slow yet steady weight loss. Do you want to give that weight loss a little gentle push? Add a little sunshine into your life.

Sunshine on Your Shoulder Makes You Happy

Have you ever heard anyone say, "I'm so sad. I feel so sunny"? Chances are, you have never heard anyone say it (unless they were being sarcastic). The sun, and its bright sunshine has always been equated to happiness or liveliness, and it is not just because of its bright yellow color.

In medicine, there is a condition known as *seasonal depression*. This is the kind of depression that results to a person being shut in without seeing the sun for a long time, such as during long stretches of winter. This kind of temporary depression is prevalent in those of older age, and in those living in countries with four seasons such as the US, but do you know the treatment for this kind of depression? You guessed it – walking outdoors during the day.

Aside from the sun producing the vitamin D precursor, sunlight also promotes the production and release of serotonin, the happy hormone. This is the hormone responsible for the feeling of elation or "high", which is sure to cure the winter blues. Walking under the sunlight only hastens the cure of the blues, as the added physical activity wakes the entire body, telling the brain that the long winter has passed.

Anytime is Good, But Early Morning is Best

So, walking, whether indoors or outdoors, whether early in the morning or in the dead of night – all of these are beneficial to the body, because you are moving, *walking*, and not being sedentary. Of course, there are conditions when a good thing can be changed to be the best, and walking outdoors in the early hours of dawn is the best time.

Now, what about *how* you should walk? What footwear should you slip on to? Should you wear flip-flops, walking shoes, or running shoes?

Chapter 4:
Grounding

When speaking to rebellious teenagers and unruly children, grounding is something of consternation, but in terms of walking, grounding is a great benefit.

Shaking the Soil Off Your Bare Feet
Earlier a question was left unanswered: should you be wearing shoes or sandals when you walk? Like the answer to when is the best time to talk a walk, wearing any of the mentioned footwear or none at all are all good for walks. However, the best thing you could do given an ideal area to walk on is to go barefoot.

Grounding or *Earthing* is a recent rediscovery—meaning this has been practiced years ago—that has caught the attention of alternative medical practitioners *and* western doctors because the benefits that grounding claims it gives the body can be backed up by science. It is an easy, natural, and free way for a person to experience the benefits of exercise while expelling toxins and further improving circulation. The first step? To step out of your shoes and onto the earth.

The principle of grounding is that we, as human beings filled with an orderly mass of wires and electrical impulses, should always be connected to the electrical grounding force that is the earth. Even in electrical engineering, grounding is a known and still-used concept to prevent static electricity from harming devices sensitive to such as well as flammable materials.

Now, this practice works in electrical engineering, but does it apply to human as well?

An Orderly Mass of Wires
Believe it or not, your body is a giant circuit, made up of smaller circuits connected with each other. The central nervous system, headed by the brain, basically fires off billions of electrical impulses in mere minutes. The heart, as well, relies on an electrical shock to jolt its chambers and valves to contract and dilate in normal sinus rhythm. In fact, if this rhythm is impaired, an artificial electrical shocker is put in place – a pacemaker.

The body contains a swirling mass of electrons from the constant exposure from all sorts of harmful radiation from electromagnetic waves, like the use and the consumption of foods cooked or heated in the microwave, mobile phones and Wi-Fi, and other things. These produce positive electrons in the body known as free radicals—the same guys you often hear about that are known to cause all sorts of problems and diseases. From what you have learned in science, opposites attract, so in order to flush out these positive electrons, you would need a strong negatively-charged element. The very earth under your feet is just that. As our bare feet come into contact with the earth (better if the earth is damp or wet, as we all know that water is a great conductor of electricity), the earth acts as a negative grounding force, freeing up the positive electrons stored in our bodies.

Disconnected

Long ago, our ancestors used to walk bare feet, or to sleep on the ground with nothing but dry grass or leaves to cover them. It might seem very squalid by today's standards, but our ancestors of old definitely had a thing going for them: they were in almost constant contact with the earth, the natural negative grounding force. They received the benefits that this rediscovered "grounding" could give, while the theory became so long forgotten as it lay buried beneath mankind's accomplishments in science and technology.

Truth be told, however, the invention of rubber or plastic soles have dealt humans more harm than anything else. Rubbers and plastics cannot conduct electricity, so all those years running on the ground or on grassy fields wearing rubber shoes did you little good. The sturdy pairs of rubber shoes, jelly flats, rubber flip-flop, plastic-soled shoes, and all other footwear have disconnected us from the earth.

It is not only our choice of footwear that disconnects us. Asphalt and wooden panels covering the soil will also block energy, so even if you walked a mile barefoot on top of a tarmac, you are still disconnected from the earth, so no grounding effect will happen.

Greatest Healer

Grounding or earthing has so many benefits that many doctors and scientists are calling it as the greatest natural healing force. Just walking along the sandy beach for half an hour or more is known to produce noticeable benefits. Have you noticed that you always seem to wake up refreshed even after a full day's activities when you are at the beach? All that time spent walking around the damp earth had you grounded, freeing you of free radicals.

Some of the known benefits of walking while grounded to the earth are:

Reduces inflammation that causes painful joints and muscles, headaches, tensions, and even chronic back pain

Improving sleeping problems such as insomnia and snoring

Increasing the body's amount of energy

Normalizing the body's circadian rhythms (the body's internal sleep cycle)

Improving blood flow and pressure

Regularizes the female menstrual cycle and reduces premenstrual symptoms

Speeds healing and even the prevention of wounds (naturalistic clinics use grounding to prevent or to treat bed sores)

Protecting and ridding the body of free radicals

Many more

Grounding or earthing is still being researched for all the benefits it brings to the body, though the above mentioned are all wonderful reasons to start walking barefoot. Many researches are still ongoing to know the full extent of the effects of earthing, but even at the early stages of research, it has been seen to be extremely promising in reducing inflammation in the body. A study being conducted tried to monitor how grounding affects body pains[3] by using heat maps to detect inflammation[4]. As there is no direct way to visualize the location and extent of pain within the body, scientists used heat as their guide instead. Inflammation causes swelling, redness, heat, and pain, so mapping out the joints and muscles that are inflamed with heat will give them visual clues.

They studied a female subject who was complaining of chronic leg and joint pain, taking note of the extent and gravity of the heat map of her lower extremities. She was subjected to a short 30-minute walk, barefoot, and the researchers found a dramatic decrease in the inflammatory heat map taken right afterwards. The heat map taken after the female test subject grounded herself showed her lower extremities displaying a lesser concentration of heated areas, as well as a lower intensity of heat, indicating that most of the inflammation has either decreased in intensity or has subsided completely. The patient herself affirmed that she felt "much better" after grounding, and that flexing her legs did not cause her as much pain as before. And this is with just 30 minutes of grounding herself! Other scientific studies are just as promising[5]!

How to Reap the Benefits

The easiest and the cheapest solution would be to take a walk on the ground, on grass (dewy grass for the best grounding benefit), dirt, rock, or at the beach without and footwear on. However, some of you might not have the luxury or the luck to have such areas nearby.

Luckily, even surfaces like concrete, ceramic tiles, and even bricks are good surfaces for grounding or earthing, so even those who are in the city will be able to benefit from it.

There are available grounding items which you can use on a daily basis, such as grounding items put into shoes or socks that will keep you grounded without having to go barefoot. There are also grounding mats where you could plant your feet onto when you are at home or at the office. However, walking while staying grounded is still the best way to achieve results, so it is highly recommended that you try this one before opting to buy items!

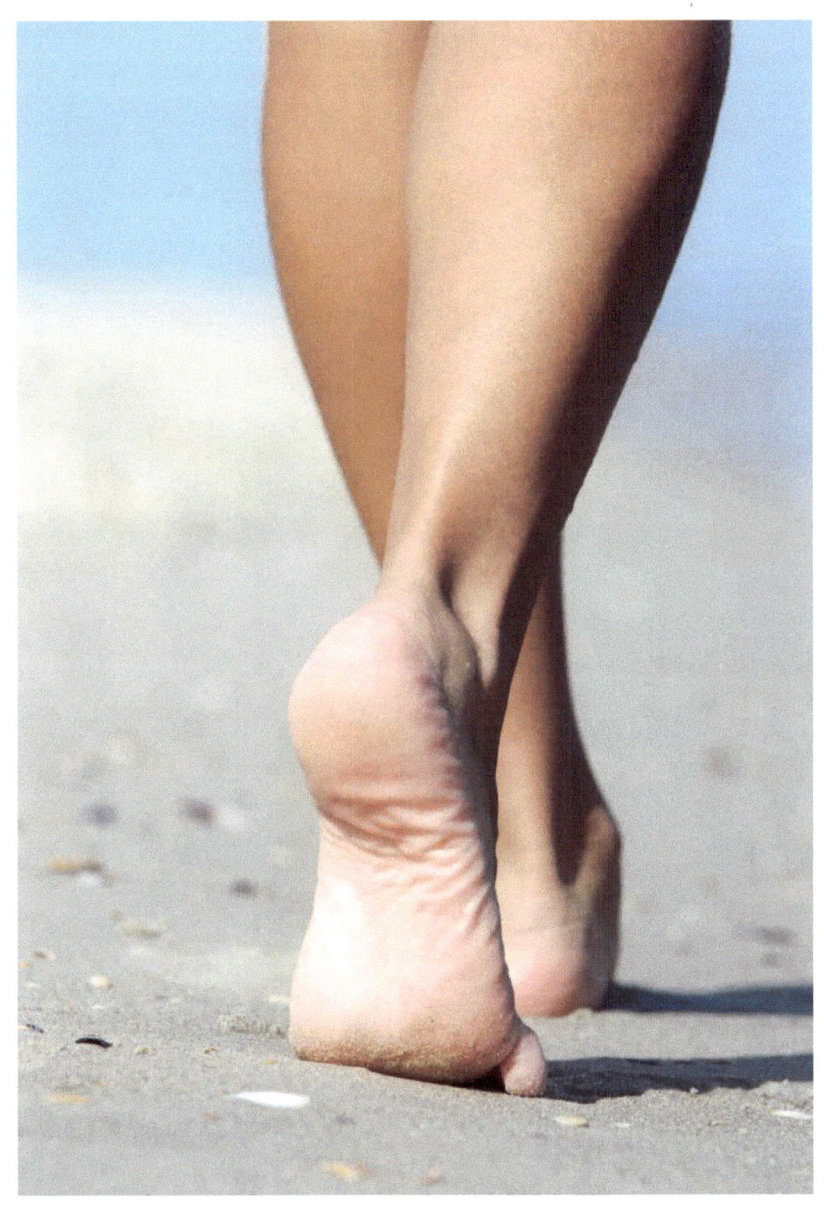

Chapter 5:
Walking in the Big Urban Jungle

Getting in tune with Mother Earth and walking miles with the feeling of live soil underneath one's bare feet is surely a wonderful thing, but sadly, not everyone is privileged enough to find a stretch of earth to walk upon in the big city. Most of you are probably living in big urban jungles, with fields of concrete and gravel instead of earth and grass. Some people are actually discouraged from getting up and walking just because of this; you might even be one of them. After all, all those facts about grounding and thalassotherapy can only work if you have regular access to the earth and sea, right?

Actually, no. you can still benefit from both of these things even when trapped in the middle of a sprawling canopy of glass and metal trees, but even putting grounding and thalassotherapy aside, the benefits of pure walking *alone* is nothing short of miraculous enough, and walking is something that no one with two working legs will have any excuse *not* to do.

Incorporating Walking into Daily Activities

If there is one thing that the invention of the treadmill desk teaches us, it is that walking is a versatile activity that can be paired up with almost anything. If you can punch numbers and type up words while walking on top of a treadmill, you can practically include walking into several aspects of your daily life, even if you are living in the big city.

Most people think of walking as plain exercise, and while it *is* a form of exercise, conditioning your mind into categorizing walking into something off-putting as exercise already gets you off the mood to do it even before you try. Many people fail to realize that above all else, walking is a mode of transportation. In fact, it was the only mode of transportation our ancestors had, eons and eons before they invented wheels. Luckily, many industrialized countries have popularized walking as a more economical form of transportation. Places like Hong Kong, Singapore, and Taiwan, for instance, encourage their urban dwellers to walk, especially if the destination is but a few blocks away. Pedestrians are given designated walk lanes so they will be safe from automobiles, and as they walk to their health, they help in reducing the volume of traffic and the amount of air pollution, too.

However, would you believe that this idea of walking as transportation did not start in the East? The practice has actually been adapted from Western countries like the US, Canada, and the UK. Yes, the practice of walking for transport originated in the big urban jungles of New York, Manhattan, and London!

Ask around your school or office and you will likely meet a person or two who regularly walks to and from the area. You could even ask them why they walk and they will tell you a number of reasons – that walking is convenient, cheaper than gas, is a good exercise, or even just to enjoy the scenery along the way. There are plenty of sound reasons to start walking, but it only takes one unwilling heart and mind to debunk all of them away.

Cutting Excuses

Finding excuses why you cannot walk is the hardest thing to overcome, because *you have already set yourself into thinking that it is something that is impossible for you to do.* If this is the case, then this section will be extremely beneficial for you, as we will throw all your excuses out the door.

1. *"I just don't have the time."*

   There are 24 hours in a day. Let us say that you use 10 hours for sleeping, 9 hours for work or school, 2 hours for daily commuting, an hour for meals, and an extra hour for chores or for relaxation. Even with such generous proportions, you *still* end up with an hour of idle time, and this is with an incredibly generous schedule!

Most people only get 5-8 hours of sleep, 8-9 hours of work or study, an hour or two of daily traffic, and two hours of daily activities. You would still get more than an hour of free time, so *there is no excuse for you not to walk for your health,* especially when you need not walk for two hours!

2. ***"I don't own a treadmill / there are no nearby gyms."***
Another petty excuse is that you don't have the equipment to start walking, such as a personal treadmill or a local gym. Firstly, you do not need treadmills or gyms to reap the benefits of walking, because you can walk practically anywhere.

This is where *walking for transportation* comes into play. You can walk to and from work or school, you can walk when you pick up your clothes at the dry cleaners, you can walk along with your dog every day. These are all good reasons to bash your "no equipment" excuse.

Secondly, do you even need a reason to go out for a walk? Why cannot walking itself *be* the reason? If you put walking at a higher priority than others, you would not be able to find excuses not to do it, but rather, find reasons *why* you should do it. If you lived in an area where walking outdoors is next to impossible, for instance, you would still reason out that walking up and down the stairs is as good as walking outside. If you do not have stairs at home, you would reason that walking inside the house is the best way to go. And if you were *really* short on space, you would still reason that marching or walking in place is better than doing nothing at all.

3. *"I don't have walking shoes at the moment."*

The beauty about walking is that it is an incredibly flexible form of exercise. You can walk as light as you want, or as robust as you want, meaning you can take it up as a serious exercise or sport, or as a light daily exercise or hobby. Like gym equipment, you do not need to have professional walking shoes to enjoy the benefits of walking. Remember grounding? In its philosophy, it is even more advisable to walk barefoot! Walking footwear are completely optional.

The important thing to note is that you should be comfortable when you walk. Whether you decide to walk barefoot or with shoes, make sure that you are comfortable, especially if you plan on walking for hours, or over long distances. You would not want to develop blisters on your soles and toes!

If you are someone who is really keen on investing in a good pair of walking shoes, however, there are a few tips in the next few chapters that you would want to take note of.

4. *"I don't have any place to walk on."*
   If you can plant your feet firmly on the ground, then you can walk. It does not matter if you are blessed to be near parks, hiking trails, or other natural areas. You can walk around the block, along the sideway, back and forth empty hallways, up and down staircases, even stationary on a treadmill or just in place in your room. The important thing is that you are off the chair and are making the motions of lifting your leg and planting one foot after another, one heel-to-toe at a time. It is this mechanical

motion that forces the pooled blood on the lower extremities to be propelled back into the circulatory system, after all, so even if you are not walking forward, you are still able to exercise your lower body effectively.

This also applies to those who find excuses not to walk because it is raining, or it is too dark, or some such. If your only free time for walking is at night, you can still make the best of it either by going to a local gym or walking inside your home.

These are but a few of the most common excuses people make to avoid walking and exercising in general. Can you hear yourself making excuses such as these? You should change the way you think about walking and of important it is in your life. Put your health into a higher priority!

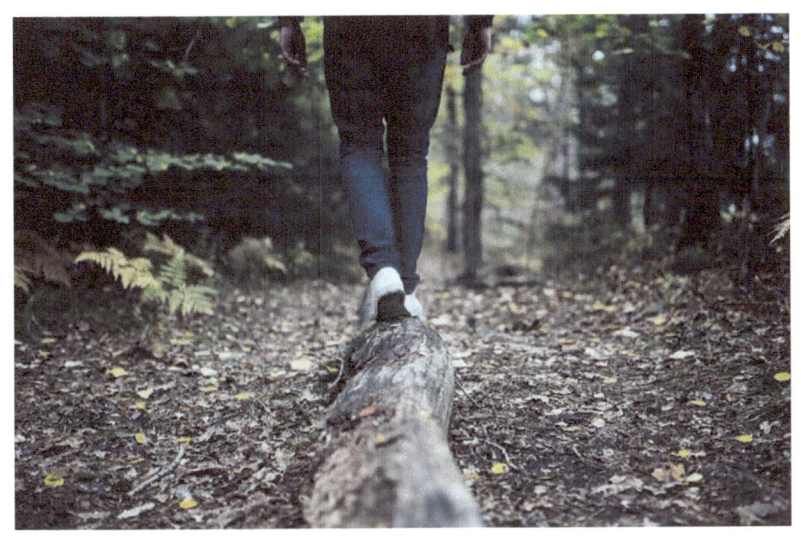

Chapter 6:
How to Get Started on Walking

Are you ready to start walking your way to a healthier body? This chapter will help you get started with a beginner's walking routine, the proper way to walk, along with some tips on how to keep you motivated in your new lifestyle.

Starting Slow

Whether you are an absolute walking neophyte or a seasoned athlete, the best way to approach any new venture is to start out slow. This will not only give you an idea of how strenuous or light an exercise you can handle, but it will also give your body the chance to pace itself accordingly. You should not feel envious or embarrassed of the other people who are power-walking their way around you – with consistent training, your body will soon adapt itself and you will gradually notice a need to progress into a more robust walking routine.

How slow is "beginner" slow? The easiest and shortest walking routine: 20 minutes. You just need to get off your chair, go out for a ten-minute walk, and walk back to your house or apartment. Simple, easy, and slow.

You should do this every day for the first week. During the week, feel yourself if you can handle this kind of exercise. Do you feel extremely tired after your walk? Is your chest painful? If this is so, you should walk even slower for the next week, and deduct 5 minutes from your walking time. This means walking out the door for 5 minutes and then heading back, for a total of 10. Do this for another week and assess yourself in the same way.

If you feel that you can accommodate a heavier exercise, you can increase the time to another 5 minutes. This means you will walk for 15 minutes, then head back for another 15, totaling to 30 minutes of walking. Do this for another week, then assess yourself. Feel free to add or subtract minutes from your routine!

Why Start Out Slow?

You might reason that since walking is such a light exercise, you could go all-out and walk a mile on your first day. This is something that is ill-advised, for a number of good reasons, with the first being that everybody's bodies are different. You could be a twenty-something college student who is otherwise healthy aside from a beer gut, or you could be a 50-something employee with diabetes and hypertension.

The body handles stress differently, depending on its current state, so what could be light exercise to one person could be beyond the capabilities of another person. Starting out in the lightest and slowest exercise is the safest course to pace your body.

A good thing to consider is that if you are one of those people who have a preexisting condition such as diabetes, hypertension, heart disease, asthma, and the like, you should consult a physician regarding your decision in starting a new exercise routine, even if it is something as light as walking. Your physician could perform stress tests to gauge your body's response to varying levels of strenuous activities, so you will have a clearer idea on what your body can handle.

Correct Posture
The best way to avoid injuries and pain after walking is to make sure that you are doing the activity correctly. Walking is such an inherent activity that most people do not realize that there is a proper way to do it.

If you stop for a moment and observe people walking along the street, you will see that there is truth in this. So many people doing the same activity, and yet there are different ways they are doing it! Some people seem to stomp the ground, while others hardly lift their feet from the floor. Others walk stiffly, hardly bending their knees, while some might shuffle or bounce about the path. Others might walk with their heads held high, hips and shoulders swinging with each confident stride, while some might slouch or droop their shoulders, their heads held low.

What is the proper way to walk? Here are a few tips:

- **Elongate your body.** Elongating your body will help stop slouching. Keep your back straight, with your head up. Your eyes should look forward.
- **Keep your shoulders back.** Your shoulders should be relaxed, not hunched up. They should be kept back and down.
- **Swing your arms.** In a relaxed walk, the arms are swinging slightly, opposite from the leg walking forward. This is natural, as this is the body's way to balance your movement.
- **Activate your stomach muscles.** Most people do not realize that most of the body's activities should involve the core muscles. Walking should not only involve just the leg muscles. You will realize how easy walking is if you let your stomach muscles in on the action. Also, most people think that "activating the core muscles" mean sucking in air and holding

it in. This is not the proper way to engage your core muscles – in fact, it is quite the opposite! If you can recall the last time you had a cough, and how your middle would hurt after days of coughing fits, you will have an idea of how to engage your core muscles. Try coughing lightly while feeling your middle – you will notice how tight it becomes. Another practice is to imagine that there is a belt around your middle and you are trying to repel that belt using just your stomach.

- **Breathe abdominally.** Another thing that most people forget is how to breathe properly. Breathing properly correlates to activating the core muscles, as the diaphragm is engaged when the core muscles are engaged. Diaphragmatic breathing is the proper way to breathe, and it is how newborns and babies breathe. However, most people revert to chest breathing when they grow up. It is quite easy to distinguish stomach breathing to chest breathing – diaphragmatic or stomach breathing inflates the stomach, while chest breathing inflates the chest. Practice stomach breathing as it is the proper and healthier way.
- **Walk with a smooth, heel-to-toe motion.** Ladies, forget what they say about the catwalk – walking is strictly a rolling heel-to-toe

motion. Your knees should be relaxed, meaning they are bent slightly and not rigidly stiff. Unlike runway advice wherein you should try walking along a straight line, putting one foot directly in front of the other, normal walking should feel more relaxed, with your feet at a regular hip-distance from each other. Also, remember to pick your feet up. There are some people who drag their feet along, or plonk their feet squarely with each stride. The correct walking motion should have a smooth rolling heel-to-toe feel. This will not only engage all the lower muscles, minimizing injuries, but will also save your footwear from unnecessary wear and tear, too.

Remember that walking should feel relaxed and natural. Women will produce a natural swinging of the hips while men will feel more comfortable with a slight swagger in the shoulders.

Choice of Footwear

If you have the opportunity to try walking barefoot along dewy grass, packed earth, smooth pavestones, bricks, or warm (but not scorching hot) concrete, please do so. Otherwise, wearing shoes or sandals is recommended, especially for those who plan on walking for longer periods.

What kind of shoes should you wear? Again, user preference is greatly considered, and it will depend on the length of your walk and the ground you will walk on. As a rule, heels are generally avoided. You would do best to stick with flat shoes like ballet flats, rubber flip-flops, or sneakers.

Rubber shoes are another popular choice, but make sure you choose the right pair. Most rubber shoes are designed for running, which, ironically, utilizes a different motion than walking. If you notice, when you are running you put most of the weight on the balls of your feet, and not the heels, so most rubber shoes have cushions along the front part of the soles. While this will provide ample shock absorbing when running, it will only hinder the natural rolling motion of ordinary walking.

Walking shoes, on the other hand, are designed specifically for the job. These shoes have cushioning and support built into the heel part of the soles, so the heels of the feet will absorb less impact. Walking shoes also have firmer arch support, allowing you a more comfortable lengthy walk.

Shoes and sneakers are recommended for harder surfaces such as wood and asphalt, though there are generally wearable in almost any terrain. Flip-flops can be quite comfortable on sand or dirt, as well as grass, but be careful to choose a pair that has a non-slip sole for wet surfaces.

Allowance and fit are also important points. Remember that when choosing a pair of shoes, the correct fit is better than something incredibly snug or too loose. If the shoes were too tight or too loose, even a simple motion such as walking will chafe the skin, causing painful blisters later on. Have your feet measured by an expert, and wear the pair around the store for a bit. Try walking around the store. Try wiggling your toes. Try standing on the tips of your toes. All these activities should be easy to do. As an added tip, you should shop for shoes in the afternoon, such as around 2-4 pm. This is the time when the feet are the largest, as they have expanded from all the early morning activities, making this time the perfect time to shop for shoes. This will ensure that the pair you will get will not turn out too tight had you bought them during the earlier hours, before the feet have had time to expand.

Generally, it is better to let the feet breathe, especially since the feet are one of the body parts that are most prone to heavy sweating. Those who would opt for flip-flops will have no problem with this, but those who would choose to wear sneakers and rubber shoes will want to wear cotton socks. You will do nicely with a pair that was designed to be breathable, too.

The Importance of Stretching

Stretching is a standard procedure before and after strenuous activities, but since walking is a very light form of exercise, you could probably skip it, right?

Wrong. You will perform any form of physical exercise best before stretching, whether it is lifting weights or walking for 15 minutes. In fact, even singers and broadcast journalists do vocalizations before performing—they are stretching their vocal muscles. Stretching conditions the muscles in anticipating a more strenuous activity to follow, so they will not be "shocked" into a sudden rigorous flexion and extension. Think of stretching as pacing your body, but on a more cellular level.

Since walking is a light exercise, however, you would not need an extensive 30-minute stretching. Simple leg, hip, and stomach stretches of around 2-3 minutes will do. Roll your hips and stomach, bend your knees, flex and extend your legs, and rotate your ankles. The ankles need more attention to avoid spraining them later on. After everything, you could do an all-body shake for 10 seconds, wherein you shake your arms and hands while lightly bouncing on your toes. This relieves the tension, helping you become more relaxed during your walk.

Staying Motivated

They say that the first step is always the hardest, but that does not mean that the second and third steps are easy. Staying motivated can be just as tough as finding that motivation to start.

A good way to stay motivated is to set goals for yourself. As a beginner, it is understandable to set lower goals, such as 1,000 steps a day, but take note that people with sedentary lifestyles average around 1,000 to 2,000 steps daily, meaning that small number might not mean much. A good beginner's goal is to take 5,000 to 10,000 steps a day. Reaching your goal will give you the drive to push on.

To help you even further, you could purchase a step counter, or a pedometer. If you have a newer-technology phone or a smartphone, you can download apps that will turn your mobile phone into your very own pedometer. You should track your normal walking rate to see how many steps you take on a regular basis. After you have an idea of this, you can set goals above your normal step rate and push yourself into reaching that goal in 2-3 days. You can then increase the goal and push yourself into reaching it again. Remember to reward yourself after every goal reached! Rewards and self-gratification will also boost your motivation.

Another great way to stay motivated is to walk with a friend or with a group. Bringing your dog, your partner, or joining a walking marathon club will be a huge help when you are feeling too stressed or lazy to continue with your walking routine. Also, the rush and elation that exercise gives is doubled when shared with other people.

If you are allergic to pets, are living alone, and have no access to walking clubs, do not fret! You can still have an invisible push through online friends and supporters. Opening up a blog dedicated to your walking progress can be a huge boost for your self-confidence and motivation, especially when others begin to respond to you. Who knows, you might even get to motivate others into taking their first step into health and wellness, too!

Lastly, positivity is a huge factor in staying motivated. If you feel positive about something, you will not let small things deter you. Starting the day with a powerful mantra like, "I will reach my goal of 4,500 steps this morning" in front of the mirror will instantly give you a huge confidence boost. This is akin to a psychological version of stretching, in which you are conditioning your mind into achieving your goal. Saying positive things will turn you positive, leading the way for a better overall experience.

Chapter 7:
Sample Walking Routine for a
Healthy Heart

At first, you might be satisfied with walking for 10-20 minutes a day. This is perfectly acceptable... for beginners. As your body adapts itself to daily light exercise, you must progress to a slightly more difficult routine until you hit the training zone that is healthy for your body, especially your heart.

The training zones are the levels of exercises that range from mild to extreme. It helps athletes and bodybuilders become more aware if their exercises are still beneficial to them or are hovering on dangerous. Different people have different safe training zones, and figuring out the safe zones mostly rely on one's measurement of one's maximum heart rate.

The heart rate is the same as the pulse, and to measure it, one has to count the number of pulses for a full minute. Activities speed up the heart rate, so it is best to take the heart rate when one is at rest, and at least an hour after eating a big meal. There are many pulse points in the body, but the easiest to feel is the one over the carotid artery, which runs along either sides of the neck. To palpate for the carotid pulse, use your index and middle fingers and gently press on the side of the neck slightly under the jawbone. You should feel a strong, clear pulse.

Keep your eyes on a wristwatch with a second hand or a wall clock and count the beats for a full minute. You may also shortcut it by counting in intervals, such as 6, 10, 20, or 30 seconds and multiplying the counted beats to a number that would make the interval into 60 (multiplied by 10 for 6 seconds, 6 for 10, 3 for 20, or 2 for 30), but of course, it is more accurate if you counted for the full minute. The normal range for the heart rate is 60-100 beats per minute, for a normal adult who is at rest. Trained athletes will normally have slower hearts, while infants and children will have normally faster-beating hearts.

Normal or at rest heart rate differs from maximum heart rate, however, in that the latter is the upper limit of what can still be considered safe in terms of exertion. To get your maximum heart rate, simply subtract your years or your age from the number 226 for women and 220 for men. The result is your maximum heart rate, meaning if your heart rate is higher than your maximum heart rate, it is considered unhealthy and even potentially dangerous.

Training zones are based on your exercising heart rate in relation to your maximum heart rate. Light exercises such as walking or warm ups, for example, are categorized as the Healthy Heart Zone, which is around 50%-60% of your maximum heart rate. So, for example that you are a man aged 42, your maximum heart rate is 178, so activities that will make your heart beat to around 89-107 beats per minute is considered light exercise.

Other training zones include the Fitness Zone, which ups your normal heart rate to about 60%-70% of your maximum heart rate; the Aerobic Zone, which ups your normal heart rate to about 70%-80% of your maximum heart rate; the Anaerobic Zone, which ups your normal heart rate to about 80%-90% of your maximum heart rate; and the Red Line Zone, which ups your normal heart rate to about 90%-100% of your maximum heart rate. For those who want walking to be their form of health maintenance exercise, training zones Healthy Heart and Fitness are both good. So, in trying to find out how fast you should walk, it will depend on how your heart will cope with the activity. Try walking normally for 10 minutes and check your pulse rate and see in which training zone it will fall under. You can then adjust your speeds accordingly, as long as your heart rate will fall under the safe training zones.

For a Healthy Heart

According to the American Heart Association, walking for at least 30 minutes a day is a good exercise to keep your heart healthy. While 30 minutes a day is a slight step up to the beginner's walking routine, once your body adjusts and strengthens itself, you will soon be able to catch up.

The AHA helped devise a 6-week walking routine for beginners who are quite getting the knack of walking for health. Their routine involves 6 days of active walking with one day of rest. Also, "walking days" have alternating or varying speeds. For example, for Monday, you will start by doing light stretches, then walk for 15 minutes. You can then rest while doing light stretches again for 2 minutes, then resume the second 15-minute walk. For Tuesday, however, there is no mandatory break in between, with you walking the full 30 minutes, though it is important to note that you should rest when your body demands it. The rest of the week alternates like this, with one day designated as the rest day.

This kind of routine goes one every day for 5 weeks, with the final sixth week bringing a bigger challenge. AHA recommends changing your pace or the speed of your walk to make the exercise heavier. In the 6th week, for instance, walkers are challenged to do power walking for one day of the week. Walkers should do the routine stretching before the exercise, then start slow by doing an easy walk for 15 minutes, then shift to bursts of 30-second power walking interspersed by a minute of easy walking, for 4-6 repetitions. Walkers should then end the exercise with the last 3-5 minutes of easy walking and a cooling down stretch.

The AHA also encourages walkers to incorporate walking into their daily routine, such as incorporating easy walking to window shopping, or including light cardio exercises while doing household chores such as cleaning windows, raking the yard, or mowing the lawn. A thing to note, however, is that you should remember to keep moving throughout window shopping or doing chores, as a prolonged sustainment of an elevated heart rate is the key in burning calories and fat.

Chapter 8:

Tips for Beneficial Walks

Now you know why walking is a wonderful thing, and also when, where, and how to walk best, here are a few more tips to make sure that your walks are as beneficial as possible!

- **Check the environment.** Walking in the city is not a new thing, but you should also take into consideration the atmospheric conditions surrounding your area and the exercise route. Check for smog, humidity, temperature, chance of rain, and the like. Have an indoor or backup plan in case of uncooperative weather conditions.
- **Map out your course.** Just because you will be just walking does not mean you can disregard checking out your walking course! You should check it out before setting out for the exercise. Check if the area is pedestrian-safe, if it is well-lighted even during the evenings, and check the condition of the terrain. You will want to take note of any uneven surfaces or holes and the like. You should also observe pedestrian traffic. Is the path heavily populated by people, people with

pets, people on bikes, or all of the above? These could potentially hinder you from having a safe and smooth walking exercise.

- **Wear sunscreen.** Even early morning light exposes you to UV rays, so remember to wear sunscreen on your face and all exposed areas a half hour before you head out. Choose a sunscreen with an SPF of no less than 30. You could also bring an umbrella, a cap, and some shades to protect yourself, especially if you are quite sensitive to light.

- **Hydrate yourself.** Walking is an exercise, and even if you decide to walk in the morning, you will still end up sweating. Remember to rehydrate yourself by drinking water before, during, and after walking. You could even bring a reusable water bottle with you. Electrolytes are also lost when sweating, so you could even eat a banana or a handful of nuts and raisins afterwards.

- **Do not push yourself.** Remember that you should pace yourself when doing physical activities, even if they are not very strenuous, like walking is. It is not advisable to walk 10 miles on your first try at walking, even if it seems easy at first glance. You do not have to push yourself – you should gradually increase the distance as your body conditions itself from the exercise.

- **Consult a physician.** This is for people who would like to try walking but are hindered or are at a disadvantage, such as people with casts, lower body weakness, or balance problems. Ask your doctor for advice so he or she could tell you what you could do.

- **Grounding without going barefoot.** Grounding or earthing can still be practiced even without having to go barefoot, but you will have to buy a small apparatus for it. It attaches to your shoe and facilitates your connection with the ground, so you can stay "grounded" even without kicking off your shoes. There are other grounding materials that you can check out, such as grounding mats that will allow you to practice grounding at home, in your office, or inside your car. Most of these items can be found online.

Conclusion

Thank you again for downloading this book!

I hope this book was able to help you realize how the simple activity of walking could provide a natural way to heal, to strengthen, and to keep the body in shape.

The next step is to kick off your shoes, knock off your socks, and try walking barefoot on the ground, just as nature intended! Try walking and grounding and you will definitely see a remarkable improvement in your health and in your daily life.

Finally, if you enjoyed this book, please take the time to share your thoughts and post a review on Amazon. It'd be greatly appreciated!

Thank you and good luck!

References and Online Resources

References

1. "The Side Effect of Sitting Down" -
    https://www.saxinstitute.org.au/media/2011-september-the-side-effect-of-sitting-down/

    "Chronic disease and sitting time in middle-aged Australian males: findings from the 45 and Up Study." -
    http://www.ncbi.nlm.nih.gov/pubmed/23394382

    "Sitting time and all-cause mortality risk in 222 497 Australian adults." -
    http://www.ncbi.nlm.nih.gov/pubmed?term=Sitting%20Time%20and%20All-Cause%20Mortality%20Risk%20in%20222%2C497%20Australian%20Adults.%20Archives%20of%20Internal%20Medicine%20201200.

2. "Cutting daily sitting time to under 3 hours might extend life by 2 years" -
    http://group.bmj.com/group/media/latest-news/cutting-daily-sitting-time-to-under-3-hours-might-extend-life-by-2-years

3. "Grounding the human body to earth reduces chronic inflammation and related chronic pain" - http://www.next-up.org/pdf/EDS_Journal_Grounding_the_human_body_to_earth_reduces_chronic_inflammation_and_related_chronic_pain_2003.pdf

4. Inflammation heat map - http://cdn2.wellnessmama.com/wp-content/uploads/earthing.jpg

5. "The Biologic Effects of Grounding the Human Body During Sleep as Measured by Cortisol Levels and Subjective Reporting of Sleep, Pain, and Stress" - http://online.liebertpub.com/doi/pdfplus/10.1089/acm.2004.10.767

   "Pilot Study on the Effect of Grounding on Delayed-Onset Muscle Soreness" - http://online.liebertpub.com/doi/pdfplus/10.1089/acm.2009.0399

Online Resources

- The Walking Site: information center on all things regarded to walking.

- American Heart Association: The 6-Week Beginner Plan for healthy walking. Also includes more advanced routines for walkers.

www.ingramcontent.com/pod-product-compliance
Lightning Source LLC
Chambersburg PA
CBHW050817290526
45792CB00001B/158